CW00521304

The Ultimate Copycat Recipes

Accurate Recipes from the Most Popular
Restaurant Meals.
Learn How Easy Can Be Cooking Like a Chef
Using the Most Common Ingredients.

JORDAN BERGSTROM

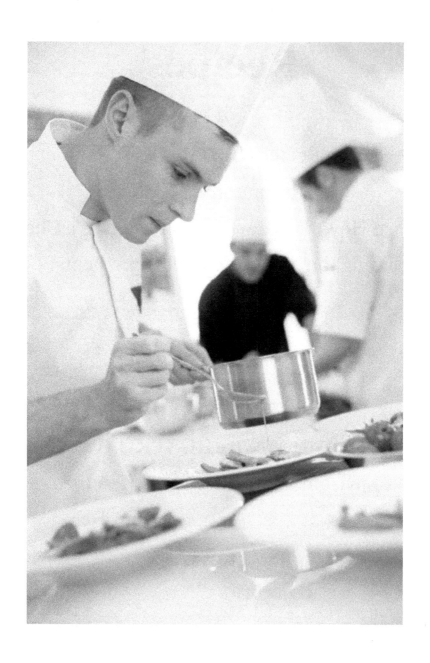

TABLE OF CONTENTS

—
4

INTRODUCTION

Thank you for purchasing this book. Copycat recipes can be so much fun to make, and this book has shown you how.

Family meals have always been a big deal at our house. There's just nothing quite like getting your friends and loved ones together in the dining room to enjoy a tasty, piping hot home cooked meal. I get that some folks love eating out, but for me, you just can't beat a home cooked meal when it comes to cost, health, and really the whole experience! But just like anyone else, I have my favorite foods that I enjoy time to time from restaurants.

There are so many reasons to be a restaurant "copycat" in the kitchen, but when the summer of 2020 hit right as I was finalizing this book, my family suddenly had a whole new reason to appreciate copycat cooking – all the restaurants (and almost everything else) were closed! Even when they reopened, the experience just wasn't the same and the safety risk hardly seemed worth it. Fortunately, with my collection of copycat recipes to rely on, the restaurant in our kitchen never closes and the menu is longer than any restaurant.

Whatever your reasons for copycat cooking, I hope you enjoy my copycat recipes. They are the product of much trial and error and each will allow you to cook a faithful representation of your favorite restaurant dishes at home.

Eating your favorite

restaurant meals at home is just one of the benefits of a copycat recipe. eat at home and save money.

Enjoy your next meal at the best restaurant in town – your dining room!

BREAKFAST RECIPES

Cracker Barrel Fried Apples

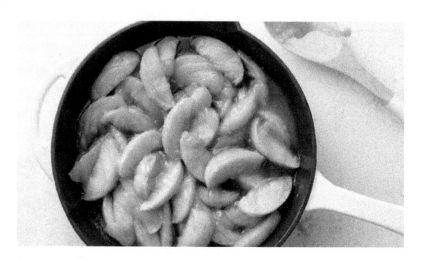

Preparation Time: 9 minutes

Cooking Time: 22 minutes

Serving: 8

Ingredients

- 8 red apples
- ¼ pound butter
- ½ cup sugar
- 1 teaspoon cinnamon
- Dash of nutmeg

Directions:

1. Do not skin the apples. Cut the apples into slices about ½" thick.
2. Cook butter in a skillet at medium heat.
3. Stir in apples and sugar to the skillet.
4. Situate lid on the skillet and cook for 20 minutes, or until the apples are tender and juicy.
5. Season with cinnamon and nutmeg before serving.

Nutrition 245 Calories 11.9g Fat 0.7g Protein

Bob Evans Sausage Gravy

Preparation Time: 11 minutes

Cooking Time: 7 minutes

Serving: 4

Ingredients

- 1-pound roll pork sausage
- ¼ cup flour
- 2 cups of milk
- Salt and black pepper, to taste
- 8 prepared biscuits

Directions:

1. Crush and cook sausage in a big skillet at medium heat until browned.
2. Mix in flour until dissolved.
3. Gradually stir in the milk.
4. Cook gravy until thick and bubbly. Cook for about 5–7 minutes, stirring constantly.
5. Season with salt and pepper.
6. Serve over hot biscuits.

Nutrition 177 Calories 11g Fat 4g Protein

Denny's Country Gravy

Preparation Time: 12 minutes

Cooking Time: 8 minutes

Serving: 4

Ingredients

- 2 tablespoons vegetable oil
- 2 tablespoons flour
- 2½ cups milk
- ¼ teaspoon salt
- ½ teaspoon pepper

Directions:

1. Cook oil and whisk in the flour.
2. Stir continuously for about 5 minutes.
3. Whisk in the milk a little simultaneously until the mixture thickens.
4. Season the gravy to taste.

Nutrition: 107 Calories 11g Fat 10.7g Protein

IHOP Harvest Grain and Nut Pancakes

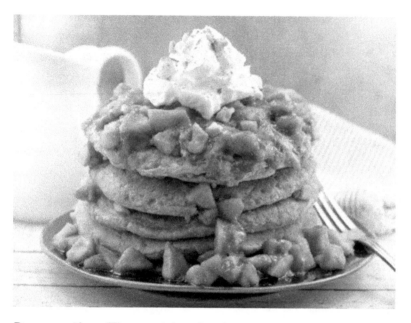

Preparation Time: 11 minutes

Cooking Time: 8 minutes

Serving: 8

Ingredients

- ¾ cup rolled oats
- ¾ cup whole-wheat flour
- 1 teaspoon baking powder
- 2 teaspoons baking soda
- ½ teaspoon salt
- 1½ cups buttermilk

- 1 egg
- ¼ cup of vegetable oil
- ¼ cup of sugar
- 3 tablespoons chopped walnuts

Directions:

1. Prep a skillet or griddle on medium heat and spray with cooking oil. Grind oats in a blender until a fine consistency.
2. Incorporate flour, oats, baking powder, baking soda, and salt. Scourge buttermilk, egg, oil, and sugar and blend with an electrical mixer until smooth.
3. Incorporate dry ingredients with the wet ingredients and blend. Add the nuts and mix.
4. Ladle 1/3 cup of batter onto a hot griddle or skillet and cook for 2–4 minutes per side.

Nutrition 202 Calories 12g Fat 5.4g Protein

McDonald's Breakfast Burrito

Preparation Time: 13 minutes

Cooking Time: 6 minutes

Serving: 4

Ingredients

- 4 ounces pork sausage
- 4 teaspoons minced onion
- ½ tablespoon minced mild green chilies
- 4 beaten eggs
- Salt and pepper, to taste
- 4 (8") flour tortillas
- 4 slices American cheese

Directions:

1. Prep a skillet over medium heat.
2. Cook sausage and onion to the skillet for 3–4 minutes.
3. Sauté chilies for 1 minute more.
4. Transfer eggs into the pan and scramble with the sausage, onion, and chilies. Season with salt and pepper.
5. Heat up tortillas in the microwave on a moist paper towel for 1 minute.

6. Transfer egg mixture and cheese to the tortilla and roll into a burrito.

Nutrition 300 Calories 16g Fat 13g Protein

McDonald's Steak, Egg, And Cheese Bagel Sandwich

Preparation Time: 12 minutes

Cooking Time: 9 minutes

Serving: 2

Ingredients

- 1 beef cube steak
- 2 tbsp. Worcestershire sauce
- 1½ tsp. garlic salt
- 1 tsp. onion
- 2 tbsp. butter
- 2 split bagels
- 2 eggs
- 2 slices American cheese

Directions:

1. Situate steaks in a plastic bag with the Worcestershire sauce, garlic salt, and onion.
2. Situate the steak on a George Foreman indoor grill for 6 minutes. Remove.
3. Grease the insides of the bagel and toast on the grill.
4. Beat the eggs in a small bowl.

5. Coat skillet with nonstick spray and cook the eggs.

6. Once set, crease in half like an omelet and slice into 4 equal pieces.

7. Situate steak on the bottom of a bagel half, add egg and cheese, then top with the other half of the bagel.

Nutrition 270 Calories 22g Fat 20g Protein

Starbucks Bran Muffins

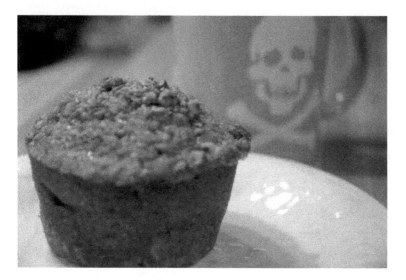

Preparation Time: 8 minutes

Cooking Time: 22 minutes

Serving: 12

Ingredients

- 2½ cups flour
- 2 teaspoons baking soda
- 1½ teaspoons salt
- 2 cups crushed bran cereal
- ½ cup chopped dried apple
- ½ cup dried cherries
- 1 cup boiling water
- ½ cup softened unsalted butter
- 1 cup sugar

- ½ cup honey
- 2 large eggs
- 2 cups buttermilk
- ½ cup walnut pieces

Directions:

1. Set oven to 400°F. Prep muffin tin with baking cups.
2. Mix flour, baking soda, and salt.
3. Scourge bran cereal and dried fruit with the boiling water.
4. In a very huge bowl, beat butter until creamy. Slowly scourge sugar, honey, and eggs.
5. Pour in buttermilk to the butter mixture and beat in. Stir in flour mixture, then bran mixture, and the walnuts.
6. Split the batter into the prepared muffin tins. Bake muffins for 20 minutes.

Nutrition 131 Calories 11g Fat 4g Protein

Bennigan's Broccoli Bites

Preparation Time: 60 minutes

Cooking Time: 7 minutes

Serving: 4

Ingredients

Broccoli Bites

- 2 cups frozen chopped broccoli
- 3 eggs
- ¾ cup shredded Colby cheese
- ¾ cup shredded Monterey jack cheese
- 5 tablespoons real bacon bits
- 1 tablespoon diced yellow onion
- 2 tablespoons flour
- 4 cups oil, for frying
- Italian breadcrumbs, as needed

Honey-Mustard Dipping Sauce

- ¾ cup sour cream
- 1/3 cup mayonnaise
- 1/3 cup Dijon mustard
- 1/3 cup honey
- 4 teaspoons lemon juice

Directions:

1. Defrost and strain broccoli thoroughly by pushing through a strainer. Scourge eggs in a mixing bowl with a whisk until well blended.

2. Situate broccoli, eggs, cheeses, bacon bits, onion, and flour into a plastic container. Blend with a spatula until thoroughly combined. Chill mixture for about 1 hour.

3. Cook 4 cups oil in a fryer or deep pan at 350°F. Situate bread crumbs in a shallow pan. Spoon a 1 tablespoon portion of the broccoli mixture into the bread crumbs. Make each portion into a ball and coat it well inside the bread crumbs.

4. Situate broccoli bites into the fry basket or frying pan. Fry for 1 minute.

5. Remove and situate onto a plate lined with paper towels to absorb excess oil.

6. For the dipping sauce, scourge sour cream, mayonnaise and mustard. Blend thoroughly using a whisk. Slowly stir in the honey and lemon juice and continue mixing until smooth and well combined. Serve with broccoli bites.

Nutrition 46 Calories 3.3g Fat 2.9g Protein

Carrabba's Bread Dipping Mix

Preparation Time: 11 minutes

Cooking Time: 0 minutes

Serving: 4

Ingredient:

- 1 tbsp. dried oregano
- 1 tbsp. dried rosemary
- 1 tbsp. dried basil
- 1 tbsp. dried parsley
- 1 tbsp. garlic powder
- 1 tbsp. black pepper
- 1 tbsp. crushed red pepper
- Salt, to taste

Directions:

1. Incorporate ingredients in a zip-top bag and crush.
2. With 1 tablespoon of the mixture in the dipping bowl.
3. Sprinkle the spices with olive oil and add a little fresh-squeezed lemon juice if desired.

Nutrition 127 Calories 14g Fat 0.1g Protein

Chili's South-Western Eggrolls

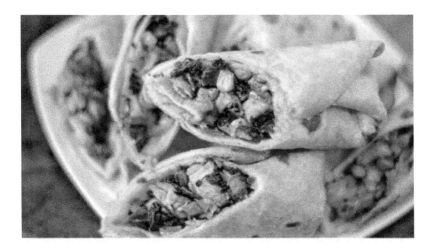

Preparation Time: 13 minutes

Cooking Time: 6 minutes

Serving: 14

Ingredient

- 1 (16-oz) can black beans
- 1 (16-oz) can drained corn
- 2 cups fresh spinach
- 2 jalapeños
- 2 garlic cloves
- ¼ cup fresh cilantro
- ¼ cup onion
- ½ tsp. chili powder
- ½ tsp. salt
- ¼ tsp. black pepper

- 2 cups Mexican cheese blend

- 15 small whole-wheat tortillas

- Prepared salsa

- Sour cream

Directions:

1. Incorporate beans, corn, spinach, jalapeños, garlic, cilantro, onion, chili powder, salt, pepper, and cheese.

2. Spread 2 tablespoons of mixture on each tortilla then roll into a thin eggroll.

3. Preheat frying pan to medium-high heat.

4. With 1 tablespoon of cooking oil per 2–3 eggrolls, shallow fry in sauté pan.

5. Garnish with salsa and sour cream.

Nutrition 132 Calories 4.4g Fat 6g Protein

APPETIZER RECIPES

Low Carb Big Mac Bites

Preparation time: 21 minutes

Cooking time: 15 minutes

Servings: 16

Ingredients:

- 1.5 pounds Ground beef
- ¼ cup Onion, finely diced
- 1 teaspoon Salt
- 4 slices American Cheese
- 16 slices Dill Pickle
- Lettuce

Secret Sauce

- 1/2 cup Mayonnaise
- 4 tablespoon Dill pickle relish
- 2 tablespoon Yellow mustard
- 1 teaspoon White wine vinegar
- 1 teaspoon Paprika
- 1 teaspoon Onion powder
- 1 teaspoon Garlic powder

Direction

1. Prep oven to 400 degrees F. Mix ground beef, onions, and salt.
2. Roll the beef into 1.5-ounce balls. Push each one down slightly to flatten it to make a mini burger patty and situate it on a lined baking sheet.
3. Bake at 400F for 15 minutes.
4. While burgers cook stir in all of the secrete sauce ingredients to a bowl and combine.
5. When done, put off the oven and remove them. Discard any excess grease off.
6. Slice each cheese slice into four squares and place a square on each mini patty. Position back in the cooling oven and let the cheese melt.
7. Place a few squares of lettuce and a pickle slice on top of each meatball then prick a skewer through it. Serve with the secret sauce and enjoy!

Nutrition 182 Calories 10g Protein 12g Fat

Keto Copycat Red Lobster Cheddar Bay Biscuits

Preparation time: 16 minutes

Cooking time: 11 minutes

Servings: 9

Ingredients:

- 1 ½ cups superfine almond flour
- ¼ tsp salt
- 1 tbsp aluminum-free baking powder
- 1 tsp garlic powder
- 2 large eggs
- 1/2 cup sour cream
- 4 tbsp unsalted butter melted
- 1/2 cup shredded cheddar cheese
- Garlic Butter Topping:
- 2 tbsp butter melted
- 1/2 tsp garlic powder
- 1 tbsp parsley minced

Direction

1. Prep oven to 450°F. Lightly coats muffin cavities of a 12-cup muffin pan.

2. Scourge almond flour, salt, baking powder, garlic powder.

3. Mix eggs, sour cream, butter. Transfer into huge bowl with dry ingredients.

4. Mix with a whisk or spoon until evenly mixed. Stir in cheese.

5. Spoon ¼ cup of batter and place into muffin mold. Repeat until all batter is used up

6. Bake biscuits about 10-11 minutes.

7. With a thin spatula to loosen edges of biscuits. Remove biscuits from muffin pan.

8. Blend garlic powder into melted butter. Stir in parsley. Brush onto tops of biscuits while the biscuits are still hot and butter is still liquid. Biscuits are best eaten warm.

Nutrition 240 Calories 7g Protein 22g Fat

Copycat Homemade Keto Bars

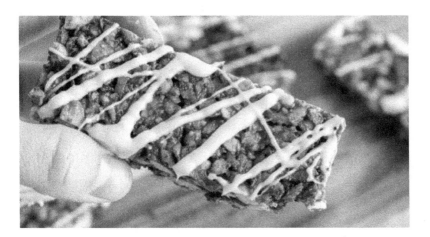

Preparation time: 12 minutes

Cooking time: 23 minutes

Servings: 6

Ingredients:

- 150 grams raw coconut meat
- 130 grams Unsweetened Bakers Chocolate
- 23 grams Unflavored Protein Powder
- 2.25 tbsp Butter
- 1.5 tbsp Water
- 3/4 tbsp Heavy Whipping Cream
- 18 grams erythritol
- 35 drops Liquid Stevia

Direction

1. Mix all the above ingredients into a food processor and combine.
2. Stop, and push all the ingredients down off the sides with a spatula and pulse again until fully immersed.
3. Create into six bars on parchment paper or into bar molds. Bake in a 250F oven for 20 minutes. Allow to cool and serve.

Nutrition 278 Calories 23g Fat 7.5g Protein

Tofu in Purgatory

Preparation time: 7 minutes

Cooking time: 21 minutes

Servings: 2

Ingredients:

- 1 tablespoon olive oil (optional)
- 2 tsp. dried herbs
- 4 large cloves of garlic
- 1 796 ml can dice tomatoes
- 1/2 teaspoon dried chili flakes
- 1 teaspoon sugar optional
- 1 block of unpressed medium tofu
- Indian Black Salt (Kala Namak) optional

Direction

1. Cook olive oil in a skillet and cook the garlic over medium heat until just starting to turn a little brown.
2. Stir in tomatoes, salt, pepper, chili flakes, herbs and optional sugar.
3. Simmer at medium heat for 5 minutes then stir the tofu rounds.

4. Put down the heat to medium-low and simmer for 15 minutes

5. Drizzle the tofu with a little Indian Black Salt just before serving if you would like an eggy flavor.

6. Serve with toast!

Nutrition 284 Calories 20g Protein 9g Fat

Keto Lemon Garlic Salmon with Leek Asparagus Ginger Sauté

Preparation time: 13 minutes

Cooking time: 22 minutes

Servings: 4

Ingredients:

For the lemon garlic salmon:

- filets of salmon (with skin on)
- 1 tbsp. (15 ml) avocado oil
- cloves garlic (12 g), minced
- teaspoons (10 ml) lemon juice
- Salt to taste
- Lemon slices to serve with

For the leek asparagus ginger sauté:

- spears of asparagus (160 g)
- 1 leek (90 g
- teaspoons (4 g) ginger powder
- Avocado oil
- 1 Tablespoon lemon juice
- Salt to taste

Direction

1. Prep oven to 400F

2. Situate each salmon filet on a piece of aluminum foil or parchment paper.

3. Split the oil, lemon juice, minced garlic between the two filets – situate these on top of the salmon. Season with some salt. Wrap up the salmon in the foil then situate into the oven.

4. Pull up the foil after 10 minutes in the oven and then bake for extra 10 minutes.

5. While cooking, situate1-2 tablespoons of avocado oil or olive oil into a frying pan and sauté the chopped asparagus and leek on high heat. Sauté for 10 minutes and then add in the ginger powder, lemon juice, and salt to taste. Sauté for 1 more minute.

6. Serve by dividing the sauté between 2 plates and placing a salmon filet on top of each.

Nutrition 680 Calories 51g Fat 43g Protein

Copycat Cauliflower Dip

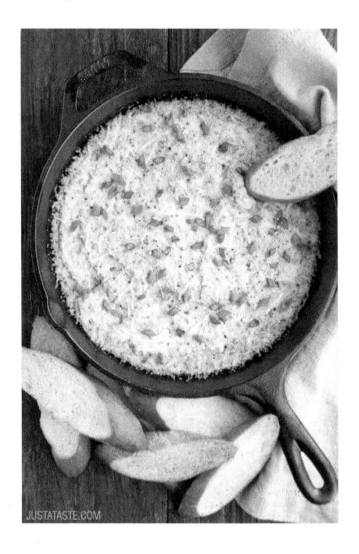

Preparation time: 11 minutes

Cooking time: 31 minutes

Servings: 2

Ingredient:

- 1/2 head of cauliflower (300 g)
- 3 Tablespoons of olive oil (45 ml)
- 3 cloves of garlic (9 g), unpeeled
- 2 Tablespoons of lemon juice (30 ml)
- Sea salt, to taste
- Radishes and cucumber sticks, to serve with

Direction

1. Prep the oven to 400°F (200°C).
2. Situate cauliflower florets in a bowl and toss with 2 tablespoons of olive oil
3. Lay them out on a prepped baking tray.
4. Get the garlic cloves as they are and secure inside a small foil parcel where no air can escape. Situate onto the same tray
5. Roast in the oven for 30 minutes, throwing the cauliflower after 15 minutes to ensure even roasting.
6. Remove the roasted, caramelized cauliflower florets and put into a mini food processor
7. Cautiously open the garlic foil parcel and squeeze the roasted flesh from the skins into the same processor. Add the lemon juice and the additional

tablespoon olive oil and blitz the mixture to a smooth puree. Season with salt.

8. Serve the roasted cauliflower dip with fresh, washed radishes and cucumber sticks, or any other vegetables you may prefer.

Nutrition 225 Calories 21g Fat 3g Protein

Creamy Cucumber Salad

Preparation time: 8 minutes

Cooking time: 0 minutes

Servings: 2

Ingredients:

- 1 cucumber (220 g), sliced and then quartered
- 2 Tablespoons of coconut cream (30 ml)
- 2 Tablespoons of lemon juice (30 ml)
- Salt, to taste

Direction

1. To make the creamy cucumber salad, mix together (in a small bowl) the cucumber slices, coconut cream, and lemon juice.
2. Add salt to taste.

Nutrition: 116 Calories 12g Fat 1g Protein

One-Bowl Keto Blueberry Muffins

Preparation time: 9 minutes

Cooking time: 23 minutes

Servings: 12

Ingredient

- 3 eggs room temp
- 1/2 cup smooth almond butter
- 2 Tbsp dairy-free milk almond
- 1/2 cup erythritol
- 2 tsp pure vanilla extract
- 1 Tbsp lemon juice
- 1 1/4 cups blanched almond flour
- 3/4 tsp baking soda
- 1/4 tsp sea salt
- 1 cup blueberries divided

Direction

1. Prep your oven to 325 and line a 12-cup muffin pan with parchment liners
2. Scourge eggs, almond butter, milk, erythritol, vanilla, and lemon juice
3. Stir in the almond flour, baking soda, and salt and mix well with a spatula or spoon, don't over-mix.

4. Mix in 2/3 of the blueberries, then scoop batter into muffin liners to make 12 muffins. Stir in remaining blueberries to the top of the batter.

5. Bake for 18-20 minutes. Set aside to cool in pan for 5 minutes, then situate to wire racks to cool completely.

6. Once cooled, serve

Nutrition 156 Calories 12g Fat 6g Protein

Copycat Grilled Eggplant and Roasted Red Pepper Dip

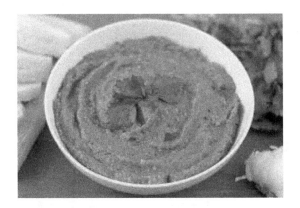

Preparation time: 12 minutes

Cooking time: 46 minutes

Servings: 6

Ingredients:

- 1 large eggplant
- 1 head garlic
- 1/2 cup diced roasted red peppers
- 2 tbsp. olive oil
- 2 tbsp. lemon juice
- 1 tbsp. fresh basil

Direction

1. Prep the grill to 400F

2. Cut top off of garlic, drizzle with olive oil, and sprinkle with sea salt. Seal in foil and situate on grill over indirect heat. Roast for 33 minutes.

3. Situate eggplant on grill and roast with lid closed, turning occasionally, for 33 minutes.

4. Cut eggplant in half and situate in colander to drain and cool. Set garlic aside to cool.

5. Peel and dice eggplant. Mesh 4 cloves of roasted garlic. Mix eggplant, mashed garlic, peppers, 3 tablespoons olive oil, lemon juice, basil, salt, and pepper. Season to taste. Drizzle of olive and fresh basil.

Nutrition 91 Calories 1g Protein 7g Fat

Roasted Garlic Baba Ghanoush

Preparation time: 12 minutes

Cooking time: 46 minutes

Servings: 6

Ingredients:

- 1 head garlic
- 2 medium eggplant
- 3- 4 tablespoons lemon juice
- 2 tbsp. tahini
- 2 tbsp. extra virgin olive oil
- ½ tsp. sea salt

Direction

1. Prep oven to 400F. Slice off the head of garlic. Situate on a sheet of foil and drizzle with olive oil. Seal tightly in foil and situate on a rimmed baking sheet with the eggplants.
2. Roast the vegetables for t 45 minutes
3. Slice eggplants in half lengthwise and situate in a colander to cool and drain. Open the garlic packet to cool.
4. Skin the eggplants and crush the flesh from the garlic head. Situate all ingredients in the food

processor and pulse to desired consistency. Taste
and adjust seasonings.

Nutrition 88 Calories 2g Protein 5g Fat

SOUPS AND BOWL RECIPES

Panera's Broccoli Cheddar Soup

Preparation Time: 15 minutes

Cooking Time: 50 minutes

Servings: 8

Ingredients:

- 1 tablespoon butter
- ½ onion, diced
- ¼ cup melted butter
- ¼ cup flour
- 2 cups milk
- 2 cups chicken stock
- 1½ cup broccoli florets, diced
- 1 cup carrots, cut into thin strips
- 1 stalk celery, sliced
- 2½ cups Cheddar cheese, grated
- Salt and pepper, to taste

Directions:

1. Cook 1 tablespoon of butter in a skillet and cook onion over medium heat for 5 minutes. Set aside.

2. In a saucepan, incorporate melted butter and flour, then cook on medium-low heat. Add 1 or 2 tablespoons milk to the meal to prevent from burning. Cook for 3 minutes.

3. While stirring, mildly pour the rest of the milk in with the flour. Stir in chicken stock. Simmer for 20 minutes. Throw in broccoli, carrots, cooked onion, and celery. Cook for an additional 20 minutes

4. Stir in cheese until melted. Sprinkle with salt and pepper, to taste.

5. Transfer into individual bowls. Serve.

Nutrition: 304 Calories 23g Fat 14g Protein

Outback's Baked Potato Soup

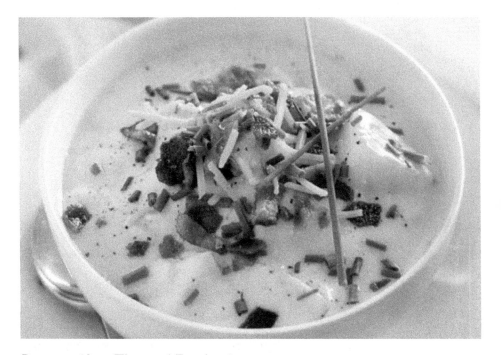

Preparation Time: 15 minutes

Cooking Time: 40 minutes

Servings: 2

Ingredients:

- 2 quarts water
- 8 medium-sized potatoes, cut into chunks
- 4 cans chicken broth
- 1 small onion, minced
- 1 teaspoon salt

- 1 teaspoon ground pepper
- 2 cups cold water
- 1 cup butter
- ¾ cup flour
- 1½ cup heavy cream
- 1½ cups jack cheese
- 2-3 thick-cut bacon slices, cooked and diced
- ¼ cup green onion, minced

Directions:

1. In a pot, fill in water and potatoes. Boil, decrease heat to medium then cook potatoes for 13 minutes. Strain and set aside.

2. In a separate pot, pour in broth and mix in onions, salt, pepper, and water. Simmer for 20 minutes.

3. Meanwhile, in another pot, whisk together butter and flour. Slowly add this to the bowl of broth. Fill in heavy cream to the mixture then simmer for 20 minutes. Mix in potatoes to reheat.

4. Drizzle jack cheese, bacon bits, and green onions on top. Serve.

Nutrition: 845 Calories 49g Fat 23g Protein

Applebee's Tomato Basil Soup

Preparation Time: 15 minutes

Cooking Time: 20 minutes

Servings: 2

Ingredients:

- 3 tablespoons olive oil
- 1 small garlic clove, finely chopped
- 1 10 ¾-ounce can condense tomato soup
- ¼ cup bottled marinara sauce
- 5 ounces water
- 1 teaspoon fresh oregano, diced
- ½ teaspoon ground black pepper
- 1 tablespoon fresh basil, diced
- 6 Italian-style seasoned croutons
- 2 tablespoons Parmesan cheese, shredded

Directions:

1. Cook oil in a pan over medium heat. Fry garlic for 2 to 3 minutes.
2. Pour tomato soup and marinara sauce into pan and stir. Add water gradually. Toss in oregano and pepper. Once simmering, reduce heat to low.

Cook for about 15 more minutes until all the flavors are combined. Add basil and stir.

3. Transfer to bowls. Add croutons on top and sprinkle with Parmesan cheese. Serve.

Nutrition: 350 Calories 26g fat 6g Protein

Chicken Enchilada Soup from Chili's

Preparation Time: 15 minutes

Cooking Time: 40 minutes

Servings: 6

Ingredients:

- 1-pound chicken breast, boneless and skinless, cut in half
- 1 tablespoon vegetable oil
- ½ cup onion, chopped
- 1 garlic clove, finely chopped
- 1-quart chicken broth
- 1 cup masa harina
- 3 cups water, divided
- 1 cup enchilada sauce
- 2 cups cheddar cheese, grated
- 1 teaspoon salt
- 1 teaspoon chili powder
- ½ teaspoon ground cumin
- Crispy tortilla strips for garnish

Directions:

1. Cook oil in a pot over medium heat. Add chicken breasts and cook evenly until browned on all sides. Remove from pot. Shred, then set aside.

2. Put pot back to heat and add onion and garlic. Sauté until onions are translucent. Add chicken broth.

3. Mix masa harina and 2 cups water in a bowl. Then, add into pot with the onions and garlic. Add the remaining water, enchilada sauce, cheddar cheese, salt, chili powder, and cumin. Bring mixture to a boil.

4. Add cooked chicken to the pot. Lower heat. Simmer for 37 minutes.

5. Garnish with crispy tortilla strips Serve.

Nutrition: 290 Calories 16g fat 22g Protein

P.F. Chang's Chef John's Chicken Lettuce Wraps

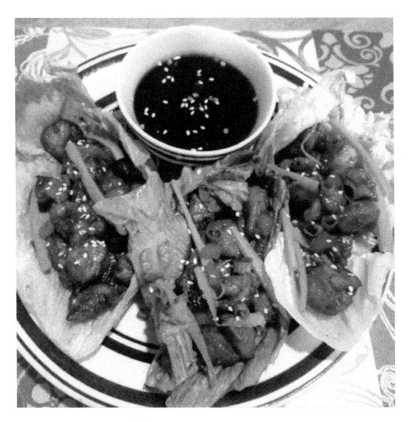

Preparation Time: 15 minutes

Cooking Time: 30 minutes

Servings: 2

Ingredients:

Chicken Mix:

- 1½ pounds skinless, boneless chicken thighs, coarsely chopped

- 1 can (8 ounces) water chestnuts, drained, minced
- 1 cup shiitake mushroom caps, diced
- ½ cup yellow onion, minced
- 1/3 cup green onion, chopped
- 1 tablespoon soy sauce
- 1 tablespoon ginger, freshly grated
- 2 teaspoons brown sugar
- 2 tablespoons vegetable oil

Glaze:

- ¼ cup chicken stock
- ¼ cup rice wine vinegar
- 4 cloves garlic, minced
- 1 tablespoon ketchup
- 1 tablespoon soy sauce
- 2 teaspoons sesame oil
- 2 teaspoons brown sugar
- ½ teaspoon red pepper flakes
- ½ teaspoon dry mustard

Herbs and Wrap:

- 1½ tablespoons fresh cilantro, chopped
- 1½ tablespoons fresh basil, chopped
- 1½ tablespoons green onion, chopped

- 16 leaves iceberg lettuce, or as needed

Directions:

1. Mix all the chicken mix ingredients (except the oil) together in a bowl. Seal with plastic wrap and situate in the refrigerator. Blend all the glaze ingredients together until everything is mixed thoroughly.

2. When the glaze is ready, cook the chicken mix ingredients in the oil over high heat.

3. After 2 minutes, when the chicken is cooked, pour half of the glaze over the chicken mix. Continue cooking the entire mixture until the glaze caramelizes. This should take 10 to 15 minutes.

4. Decrease heat to medium to low, then add the remaining glaze to the mixture. Cook for around 3 more minutes, continually stirring.

5. Stir in the chopped herbs and continue cooking until they are incorporated into the chicken mixture.

6. Situate the chicken to a plate and serve with lettuce.

Nutrition: 212 Calories 11g Fat 18g Protein

Apple Walnut Chicken Bowl

Preparation Time: 15 minutes

Cooking Time: 30 minutes

Servings: 2

Ingredients:

For the chicken

- 3 cups water
- 1 tablespoon salt
- ½ teaspoon garlic powder
- ¼ teaspoon hickory-flavored liquid smoke
- 1 boneless chicken breast, pounded to ½-inch thickness
- ½ teaspoon ground black pepper
- 1 tablespoon oil

For the balsamic vinaigrette

- ¼ cup red wine vinegar
- 3 tablespoons granulated sugar
- 3 tablespoons honey
- 1 tablespoon Dijon mustard
- ½ teaspoon salt
- 1 teaspoon minced garlic
- 1 teaspoon lemon juice

- ½ teaspoon Italian seasoning
- ¼ teaspoon dried tarragon
- Pinch ground black pepper
- 1 cup extra-virgin olive oil
- For the candied walnuts
- 1 teaspoon peanut oil
- 1 teaspoon honey
- 2 tablespoons granulated sugar
- ¼ teaspoon vanilla extract
- 1/8 teaspoon salt
- Pinch cayenne pepper
- ¾ cup chopped walnuts

For the salad

- 4 cups romaine lettuce, chopped
- 4 cups red leaf lettuce, chopped
- 1 apple, diced
- ½ small red onion, sliced
- ½ cup diced celery
- ¼ cup blue cheese, crumbled

Directions:

For the chicken brine

1. Mix together the water, salt, garlic powder, and liquid smoke in a medium-sized bowl.
2. Stir in chicken, cover, and chill for three hours.
3. For the balsamic vinaigrette
4. Whisk together all ingredients listed EXCEPT the oil.
5. Gradually pour in the oil while whisking. Refrigerate until ready to serve.

For the candied walnuts

1. In a skillet, mix together the peanut oil, honey, sugar, vanilla, salt, and cayenne pepper, and cook over medium heat.
2. Once it starts to boil, drizzle in the walnuts and stir until the sugar begins to caramelize. Stir for 1 minute then pour onto a baking sheet covered with wax paper. Allow the nuts to cool.

For the salad

1. Pull out the chicken from the brine and pat it dry with paper towel. Season with black pepper.
2. Place the chicken on a hot grill. Grill for 8 minutes on both sides. Allow to cool and chop it into strips.
3. In a salad bowl, combine the romaine lettuce, red leaf lettuce, apple, onion, celery, and blue

cheese. Divide it onto plates and pour on some dressing. Top with sliced chicken and candied walnuts.

4. Refrigerate any unused dressing.

Nutrition: 402 Calories 21g Fat 34g Protein

Cheesy Walkabout Soup

Preparation Time: 15 minutes

Cooking Time: 50 minutes

Servings: 2

Ingredients:

- 6 tablespoons butter, divided
- 2 large sweet onions, thinly sliced
- 2 cups low sodium chicken broth
- ¼ teaspoon ground black pepper
- 2 chicken bouillon cubes
- 3 tablespoons flour
- ¼ teaspoon salt
- 1 ½ cups whole milk
- Pinch nutmeg
- ¼ cup Velveeta® cheese, cubed

Direction:

1. Using Dutch oven, melt half the butter over medium heat. Cook onions, stirring irregularly, until transparent but not browned.
2. Add the chicken broth, black pepper, and bouillon cubes. Mix well and cook on low to heat through.

3. In a separate saucepan, melt the remaining butter. Add the flour and salt and cook, whisking constantly, until smooth and lightly browned. Slowly whisk in the milk and cook at medium heat until it is very thick. Mix in the nutmeg.

4. Add the white sauce to the onion soup mixture, together with the Velveeta cubes. Stir gently over medium heat until the cheese is melted, and everything is combined.

Nutrition: 260 Calories 19g Fat 5g Protein

Roasted Red Pepper Soup

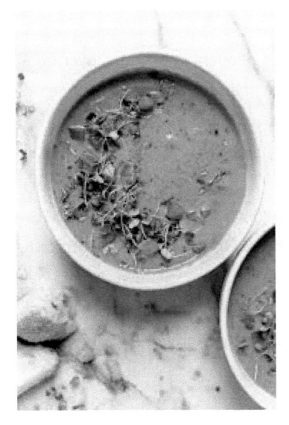

Preparation Time: 15 minutes

Cooking Time: 40 minutes

Servings: 8

Ingredients:

- 1-pound cauliflower rice or cauliflower, chopped
- 2-1/2 pounds sweet peppers
- 1-1/2 tsp. sweetener
- 2 cups half and half

- 1-1/2 tsp. salt
- 2 cups chicken or vegetable broth

Directions

1. Arrange the sweet peppers in a single layer on a large-sized baking sheet & roast until softened & browned slightly, for half an hour, at 400 F.
2. In the meantime, add the broth & cauliflower to a large stock pot. Let simmer until the peppers are done, over medium heat settings.
3. Add in the cauliflower, peppers, half the broth & the leftover ingredients to a blender. Blend until creamy, for 2 minutes. Add the mixture to the pot again & cook until heated through

Nutrition: 305 Calories 5g Fat 34g Protein

Chili's Chili

Preparation Time: 10 minutes

Cooking Time: 1 hour and 10 minutes

Servings: 8

Ingredients:

For Chili:

- 4 pounds ground chuck - ground for chili
- 1 ½ cups yellow onions, chopped
- 16 ounces tomato sauce
- 1 tablespoon cooking oil
- 3 ¼ plus 1 cups water
- 1 tablespoon masa harina

For Chili Spice Blend:

- 1 tablespoon paprika
- ½ cup chili powder
- 1 teaspoon ground black pepper
- 1/8 cup ground cumin
- 1 teaspoon cayenne pepper or to taste
- 1/8 cup salt
- 1 teaspoon garlic powder

Directions:

1. Combine the entire chili spice ingredients together in a small bowl; continue to combine until thoroughly mixed.

2. Now, over moderate heat in a 6-quart stock pot; place & cook the meat until browned; drain. In the meantime; combine the chili spice mix together with tomato sauce & 3 ¼ cups of water in the bowl; give the ingredients a good stir until blended well.

3. Add the chili seasoning liquid to the browned meat; give it a good stir & bring the mixture to a boil over moderate heat.

4. At medium heat in a big skillet; cook 1 tablespoon of the cooking oil & sauté the onions until translucent, for a couple of minutes. Add the sautéed onions to the chili.

5. Decrease the heat to low & let simmer for an hour, stirring after every 10 to 15 minutes. Combine the masa harina with the leftover water in a separate bowl; mix well. Add to the chili stock pot & cook for 10 more minutes.

Nutrition: 205 Calories 5g Fat 34g Protein

Enchilada Soup

Preparation Time: 10 minutes

Cooking Time: 15 minutes

Servings: 10

Ingredients:

- 2 rotisserie chickens or 3 pounds cooked diced chicken
- ½ pound processed American cheese
- 3 cups yellow onions, diced
- ¼ cup chicken base
- 2 cups masa harina
- ½ teaspoon cayenne pepper
- 2 teaspoon granulated garlic
- 1 teaspoons salt
- 2 cups tomatoes, crushed
- ½ cup vegetable oil
- 2 teaspoon chili powder
- 4 quarts water
- 2 teaspoon ground cumin

Directions:

1. Over moderate heat in a large pot; combine oil together with onions, chicken base, granulated

garlic, chili powder, cumin, cayenne & salt. Cook for 3 to 5 minutes, until onions are soft & turn translucent, stirring occasionally.

2. Combine 1 quart of water with masa harina in a large measuring cup or pitcher.

3. Continue to stir until no lumps remain. Add to the onions; bring the mixture to a boil, over moderate heat.

4. Once done, cook for a couple of minutes, stirring constantly. Stir in the tomatoes & leftover 3 quarts of water. Bring the soup to a boil again, stirring every now and then. Add in the cheese.

5. Cook until the cheese is completely melted, stirring occasionally. Add the chicken & cook until heated through. Serve immediately & enjoy.

Nutrition: 105 Calories 5g Fat 34g Protein

MAIN RECIPES

Wendy's Apple Pecan Salad with Chicken

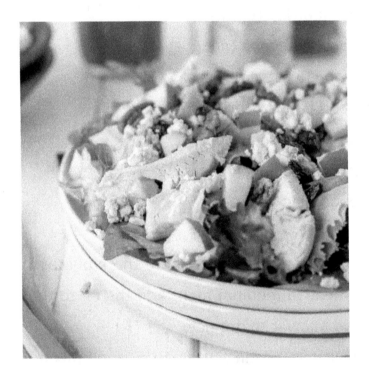

Preparation Time: 9 minutes

Cooking Time: 10 minutes

Serving: 3

Ingredients:

- 2 tablespoons vegetable oil
- 2 chicken breasts
- 2 cups Romaine lettuce
- 1 cup spinach
- ¼ cup strawberries (sliced)
- ¼ cup cranberries (dried)
- 2 tablespoons pecans (chopped)
- ½ cup bleu cheese crumbles
- ¼ teaspoon parsley (dried)
- ¼ teaspoon garlic powder
- ¼ teaspoon Himalayan sea salt
- ¼ teaspoon black pepper

Directions:

1. Place a medium-sized skillet onto the stove and turn the heat to medium high. Add the oil to the skillet and allow it to get hot.
2. As the skillet is heating up, take a small mixing bowl and add the garlic powder, parsley, sea salt, and black pepper. Stir until well combined.
3. Take each of the chicken breasts and sprinkle on the garlic powder mixture on all sides.

4. Place your seasoned chicken breast into the skillet. Cook the chicken for five minutes then flip and cook for another five minutes. Once the internal temperature of the chicken has reached 165 degrees Fahrenheit, remove from the skillet and allow it to rest on a cutting board.

5. While resting, prep the rest of your salad. In a big salad bowl add the spinach, lettuce, strawberries, and cranberries. Toss everything together with salad spoons. Divide the salad into two equal portions and top each portion with half the pecans and bleu cheese.

6. Slice the chicken breast and place on top of your salad. Serve with your preferred keto-friendly salad dressing.

Nutrition 538 Calories 46g Fat 24g Protein

P.F. Chang's Chicken Lettuce Wraps

Preparation Time: 13 minutes

Cooking Time: 21 minutes

Serving: 4

Ingredients:

- 1 tablespoon avocado oil
- 1-pound chicken (ground)
- 1 head of butter lettuce
- 2 cups shiitake mushrooms (chopped)
- 3 green onions (sliced)
- ½ cup jicama (diced)
- 2 teaspoons onion powder
- ¼ teaspoon Himalayan sea salt
- ¼ teaspoon black pepper

For Sauce:

- 1 tablespoon sesame oil
- 2 cloves of garlic (minced)
- ½ teaspoon ginger (grated)
- ½ tablespoon erythritol (sweetener)
- 3 tablespoons coconut amino
- 1 tablespoon apple cider vinegar
- 1 tablespoon almond butter

Directions:

1. Begin by making the sauce first. Using a medium-sized mixing bowl, mix sesame oil, minced garlic, grated ginger, erythritol, coconut amino, apple cider vinegar, and almond butter. Use a whisk to vigorously mix everything together. Cover and store in your refrigerator until ready.

2. Now, take a large skillet and place it on your stove with a tablespoon of avocado oil in it. Turn the heat to medium, so the oil can get nice and hot. When the oil is heated, add in your ground chicken. Use a spatula to break it apart as it cooks. Allow the chicken to cook for 8 minutes or until it has all turned a light brown color.

3. Once cooked, stir in the onion powder, sea salt, and black pepper. Stir everything together then add in the shiitake mushrooms, green onions, and jicama. Stir and cook for 5 minutes.

4. Once the mushrooms have softened, after about 5 minutes, pour your sauce over the top. Let the mixture simmer for 5 minutes then turn off the heat.

5. Take you butter lettuce and carefully remove the leaves. Place a leaf on a plate and spoon a quarter cup of the chicken mixture in the center. Repeat until you have used up the chicken mixture. Serve and enjoy!

Nutrition 155 Calories 5g Fat 18g Protein

In-N-Out Burger

Preparation Time: 8 minutes

Cooking Time: 13 minutes

Serving: 4

Ingredients:

- 1 ½ pounds lean ground beef
- 5 slices cheddar cheese
- 20 lettuce leaves
- 1 teaspoon Himalayan sea salt
- 1 teaspoon black pepper

optional toppings:

- tomato slices
- onion slices
- pickle slices

For the Sauce:

- ½ cup mayonnaise
- 1 tablespoon sugar-free ketchup
- 1 teaspoon mustard paste
- 2 tablespoons pickles (diced)
- 2 teaspoon pickle juice
- ½ teaspoon paprika
- ½ teaspoon garlic powder

- ½ teaspoon Himalayan sea salt

Directions:

1. Begin by preparing the sauce. Combine the mayonnaise, sugar-free ketchup, mustard paste, diced pickles and pickle juice, paprika, garlic powder, and sea salt into a medium mixing bowl. Whisk everything together thoroughly, cover the bowl with plastic wrap, and store in the refrigerator until ready.

2. Next, you want to place a griddle pan or grill pan on your stove. Add a little bit of oil or cooking spray to the pan and turn the heat to medium, so it gets nice and hot as you prepare your patties.

3. In a large mixing bowl, add your ground beef, sea salt, and black pepper. Use your hands to mix everything together. Portion out the meat into five equal servings and roll them into a ball form then flatten slightly to form your patties. Place your patties onto your hot griddle and cook for 5 minutes on each side or until they turn a dark brown color.

4. When the burgers are done cooking, turn the heat off the stove and top the patties with your cheddar cheese slices.

5. To assemble your patties, lay two leaves of lettuce down first. Place your burger patty on the lettuce leaf, top with your favorite burger toppings, then take the sauce you prepared early and drizzle it over top. Place another two lettuce leaves on top and enjoy!

Nutrition 466 Calories 26g Fat 49g Protein

Buffalo Wild Wings Spicy Garlic Sauce Chicken Wings

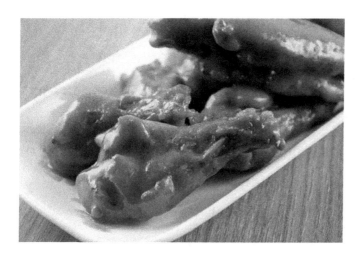

Preparation Time: 13 minutes

Cooking Time: 50 minutes

Serving: 4

Ingredients:

- 2 ½ pounds chicken wings
- ½ teaspoon Himalayan sea salt

For Sauce:

- ¼ cup avocado oil
- ½ cup hot sauce
- 2 tablespoons garlic powder
- ¼ teaspoon cayenne pepper

- ½ teaspoon Stevia (liquid)

Direction:

1. Prep your oven to 400 degrees Fahrenheit.
2. Pat-dry your wings with a paper towel then situate them on a wire rack. Season them with sea salt and place them in the oven for 45 minutes.
3. After 45 minutes, adjust oven to broil and keep the wings in your oven for an extra 5 minutes
4. Blend the avocado oil, hot sauce, garlic powder, cayenne pepper, and liquid stevia in a blender until you have a smooth mixture then transfer to a large mixing bowl
5. When the wings have come out of the oven, situate them into the bowl with your sauce. Throw the wings so that they all get generously coated.

Nutrition 466 Calories 26g Fat 49g Protein

Chick-Fil-A's Chicken Nuggets

Preparation Time: 2 hours

Cooking Time: 21 minutes

Serving: 4

Ingredients:

- 2 eggs
- 2 tablespoons heavy cream
- 1-pound chicken breast (cut into 1-inch pieces)
- 1 ½ cups panko breadcrumbs
- ½ cup pickle juice
- ½ teaspoon garlic powder
- ¼ teaspoon paprika
- ½ teaspoon Himalayan sea salt
- ¼ teaspoon black pepper

Directions:

1. Place your 1-inch cut chicken pieces into a sealable plastic bag. Pour in the pickle juice, seal the bag, and shake to ensure the chicken is well coated with the juice. Situate bag into the refrigerator for 2 hours.

2. When ready, preheat your oven to 425 degrees Fahrenheit. Then, line a baking sheet with parchment paper. Set the baking sheet to the side.

3. Take a medium-sized mixing bowl and combine the panko breadcrumbs, garlic powder, paprika, sea salt, and black pepper. With a fork to mix everything together, then transfer to a sealable plastic bag and set to the side.

4. Take another medium-sized bowl and crack your eggs into it. Add in the heavy cream and beat together with a fork. Take your chicken pieces out of the refrigerator and transfer into the egg mixture. Make sure each piece gets well coated with the egg mixture.

5. Next, use tongs to transfer the chicken from the egg mixture to the plastic bag with the breadcrumbs. Give the bag a few shakes and gently press the breadcrumbs into the chicken pieces. When the chicken looks evenly coated, remove them from the bag and place them on a roasting rack set on top of your lined baking

sheet. Situate chicken into the oven and bake for 20 minutes.

6. Once the chicken is a crispy golden color remove from the oven and serve.

Nutrition 261 Calories 9.5g Fat 45g Protein

PASTA AND PIZZA RECIPES

Greek Olive and Feta Cheese Pasta

Preparation Time: 90 Minutes

Cooking Time: 15 Minutes

Servings: 2

Ingredients:

- 2 cloves of finely minced fresh garlic
- 2 large tomatoes, seeded and diced
- 3 oz. feta cheese, crumbled
- ½ diced red bell pepper
- 10 small-sized Greek olives, coarsely chopped and pitted
- ½ diced yellow bell pepper
- ¼ cup basil leaves, coarsely chopped
- 1 Tbsp. Olive oil
- ¼ tsp. hot pepper, finely chopped
- 4 ½ oz. of ziti pasta

Directions:

1. Cook pasta to a desirable point, drain it, sprinkle with olive oil, and set aside.
2. In a large bowl, mix olives, feta cheese, basil, garlic, and hot pepper. Leave for 30 minutes.
3. To the same bowl, add the cooked pasta, the bell peppers, and toss. Refrigerate for up to an hour. Toss again, then serve chilled.

Nutrition: Calories: 235 kcal Carbs: 27g Fat: 10g Protein: 7g.

Eggs with Zucchini Noodles

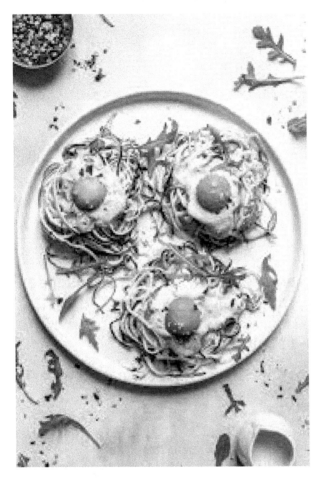

Preparation Time: 10 Minutes

Cooking Time: 11 Minutes

Servings: 2

Ingredients:

- 2 tablespoons extra-virgin olive oil
- 3 zucchinis, cut with a spiralizer

- 4 eggs
- Salt and black pepper to the taste
- A pinch of red pepper flakes
- Cooking spray
- 1 tablespoon basil, chopped

Directions:

1. In a plate, combine the zucchini noodles with salt, pepper and the olive oil and toss well.
2. Grease a baking sheet by means of cooking spray and divide the zucchini noodles into 4 nests on it.
3. Crack an egg on each nest, sprinkle salt, pepper and the pepper flakes on top then bake at 350 degrees F for 11 minutes.
4. Divide the mix between plates, sprinkle the basil on top and serve.

Nutrition: Calories: 296 Protein: 15 g Fat: 24 g Carbs: 11 g

Portobello Mushroom Pizza

Preparation Time: 20 Minutes

Cooking Time: 12 Minutes

Servings: 4

Ingredients:

- ½ teaspoon red pepper flakes
- A handful of fresh basil, chopped
- 1 can black olives, chopped
- 1 medium onion, chopped
- 1 green pepper, chopped
- ¼ cup chopped roasted yellow peppers
- ½ cup prepared nut cheese, shredded
- 2 cups prepared gluten-free pizza sauce
- 8 Portobello mushrooms, cleaned and stems removed

Directions:

1. Preheat the oven toaster.
2. Take a baking sheet and grease it. Set aside.
3. Place the Portobello mushroom cap-side down and spoon 2 tablespoons of packaged pizza sauce on the underside of each cap. Add nut cheese and top with the remaining ingredients.

4. Broil for 12 minutes or until the toppings are
   wilted.

Nutrition: Calories per Serving: 578 Carbs: 73.0g
Protein: 24.4g Fat: 22.4g

Cajun Garlic Shrimp Noodle Bowl

Preparation Time: 15 Minutes

Cooking Time: 15 Minutes

Servings: 2

Ingredients:

- ½ teaspoon salt
- 1 onion, sliced
- 1 red pepper, sliced
- 1 tablespoon butter
- 1 teaspoon garlic granules
- 1 teaspoon onion powder
- 1 teaspoon paprika
- 2 large zucchinis, cut into noodle strips
- 20 jumbo shrimps, shells removed and deveined
- 3 cloves garlic, minced
- 3 tablespoon ghee
- A dash of cayenne pepper
- A dash of red pepper flakes

Directions:

1. Prepare the Cajun seasoning by mixing the onion powder, garlic granules, pepper flakes, cayenne

pepper, paprika, and salt. Toss in the shrimp to coat in the seasoning.

2. In a skillet, heat the ghee and sauté the garlic. Add in the red pepper and onions and continue sautéing for 4 minutes.
3. Add the Cajun shrimp and cook until opaque. Set aside.
4. In another pan, heat the butter and sauté the zucchini noodles for three minutes.
5. Assemble by placing the Cajun shrimps on top of the zucchini noodles.

Nutrition: Calories per Serving: 712 Fat: 30.0g Protein: 97.8g Carbs: 20.2g

Pasta with Peas

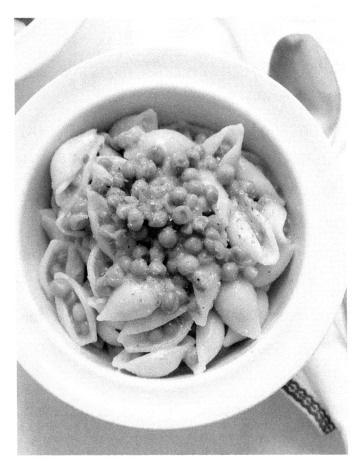

Preparation Time: 10 Minutes

Cooking Time: 10 Minutes

Servings: 4

Ingredients:

- 2 eggs
- 1 cup frozen peas
- ½ cup Parmigiano-Reggiano cheese, grated

- 12 ounces linguini
- 1 Tbsp. olive oil
- 1 onion, sliced
- Salt & pepper, to taste

Directions:

1. In a dish, combine the zucchini noodles with salt, pepper and the olive oil and toss well.
2. Prepare linguini according to the package.
3. Whisk eggs and mix in cheese.
4. Sauté onion in olive oil, then stir in peas. Add pasta to pan.
5. Add egg mixture to the pasta and cook for another 2 min. Season with salt and pepper.
6. Serve hot.

Nutrition: Calories: 480 Protein: 20 g Fat: 11 g Carbs: 73 g

DESSERT RECIPES

Chocolate Pudding Delight

Preparation Time: 52 minutes

Cooking Time: 0 minutes

Servings: 2

Ingredients:

- 1/2 teaspoon stevia powder
- 2 tablespoons cocoa powder
- 2 tablespoons water
- 1 tablespoon gelatin
- 1 cup of coconut milk
- 2 tablespoons maple syrup

Directions:

1. Heat the pan with the coconut milk over medium heat; add stevia and cocoa powder and mix well.
2. In the bowl, mix gelatin with water, stir well and add to the pan.
3. Stir well, add maple syrup, whisk again, divide into ramekins and keep in the fridge for 45 minutes. Serve cold.

Nutrition: 221 Calories 14g Fat3.4g Protein

Cinnamon Streusel Egg Loaf

Preparation Time: 10 minutes

Cooking Time: 15 minutes

Servings: 2

Ingredients:

- 2 tbsp. almond flour
- 1 tbsp. butter softened
- ½ tbsp. grated butter, chilled
- 1 egg
- 1-ounce cream cheese

Others:

- ½ tsp cinnamon, divided
- 1 tbsp. erythritol sweetener, divided
- ¼ tsp vanilla extract, unsweetened

Directions:

1. Turn on your oven and then set it to 350 degrees F and let it preheat.
2. Meanwhile, crack the egg in a small bowl, add cream cheese, softened butter, ¼ tsp cinnamon,

½ tbsp. Sweetener and vanilla and whisk until well combined.

3. Divide the egg batter between two silicone muffins and then bake for 7 minutes.

4. Meanwhile, prepare the streusel and for this, place flour in a small bowl, add remaining ingredients and stir until well mixed.

5. When egg loaves have baked, sprinkle streusel on top and then continue baking for 7 minutes.

6. When done, remove loaves from the cups, let them cool for 5 minutes and then serve and enjoy!

Nutrition: 152 Calories 15g Fats 4g Protein

Snickerdoodle Muffins

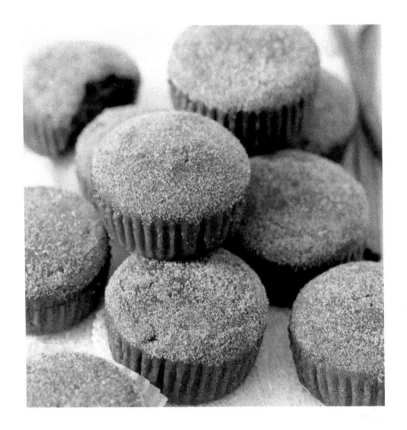

Preparation Time: 10 minutes

Cooking Time: 12 minutes

Servings: 2

Ingredients:

- 6 2/3 tbsp. coconut flour
- ½ of egg
- 1 tbsp. butter, unsalted, melted
- 1 1/3 tbsp. whipping cream

- 1 tbsp. almond milk, unsweetened

Others:

- 1 1/3 tbsp. erythritol sweetener and more for topping
- ¼ tsp baking powder
- ¼ tsp ground cinnamon and more for topping
- ¼ tsp vanilla extract, unsweetened

Directions:

1. Turn on the oven, then set it to 350 degrees F and let it preheat.
2. Meanwhile, take a medium bowl, place flour in it, and add cinnamon and baking powder. Stir until combined.
3. Take a separate bowl, place the half egg in it, add butter, sour cream, milk, and vanilla and whisk until blended.
4. Whisk in flour mixture until a smooth batter is obtained, divide the batter evenly between two silicon muffin cups and then sprinkle cinnamon and sweetener on top.

5. Bake the muffins for 10 to 12 minutes until firm, and then the top has turned golden brown and then serve and enjoy!

Nutrition: 241 Calories 21g Fats 7g Protein

Yogurt and Strawberry Bowl

Preparation Time: 5 minutes

Cooking Time: 0 minutes

Servings: 2

Ingredients:

- 3 oz. mixed berries
- 1 tbsp. chopped almonds
- 1 tbsp. chopped walnuts
- 4 oz. yogurt

Directions:

1. Divide yogurt between two bowls, top with berries and then sprinkle with almonds and walnuts.
2. Serve and enjoy!

Nutrition: 165 Calories 11g Fats 9.3g Protein

Sweet Cinnamon Muffin

Preparation Time: 5 minutes

Cooking Time: 2 minutes

Servings: 2

Ingredients:

- 4 tsp coconut flour
- 2 tsp cinnamon
- 2 tsp erythritol sweetener
- 1/16 tsp baking soda
- 2 eggs

Directions:

1. Take a medium bowl, place all of the ingredients in it, & whisk until well combined.
2. Take two ramekins, grease them w/ oil, distribute the prepared batter in it & then microwave for 1 min. & 45 secs. Until done.
3. When done, take out muffin from the ramekin, cut in half, & then serve and enjoy!

Nutrition: 101 Calories 7g Fats8g Protein

Nutty Muffins

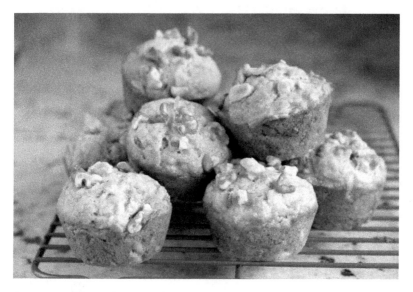

Preparation Time: 5 minutes

Cooking Time: 5 minutes

Servings: 2

Ingredients:

- 4 tsp coconut flour
- 1/16 tsp baking soda
- 1 tsp erythritol sweetener
- 2 eggs
- 2 tsp almond butter, unsalted

Directions:

1. Take a medium bowl, place all the ingredients in it, and whisk until well combined.

2. Take two ramekins, grease them with oil, distribute the prepared batter in it & then microwave for 1 minute and 45 seconds until done.
3. When done, take out muffin from the ramekin, cut in half, and then serve and enjoy!

Nutrition: 131 Calories 8.6g Fats 8g Protein

Pumpkin and Cream Cheese Cup

Preparation Time: 10 minutes

Cooking Time: 12 minutes

Servings: 2

Ingredients:

- 4 tbsp. almond flour
- 1 1/3 tbsp. coconut flour
- 2 tbsp. pumpkin puree
- 2 2/3 tbsp. cream cheese softened
- ½ of egg
- 2/3 tbsp. butter, unsalted
- ¼ tsp pumpkin spice
- 2/3 tsp baking powder
- 2 tbsp. erythritol sweetener

Directions:

1. Turn on the oven, then set it to 350 degrees F & let it preheat.
2. Take a medium bowl, place butter, and 1 ½ tbsp. The sweetener in it, and then beat until fluffy.
3. Beat in egg and then beat in pumpkin puree until well combined.

4. Take a medium bowl, place flours in it, stir in pumpkin spice, baking powder until mixed, stir this mixture into the butter mixture and then distribute it into two silicone muffin cups.

5. Take a medium bowl, place cream cheese in it, and stir in remaining sweetener until well combined.

6. Divide the cream cheese mixture into the silicone muffin cups, swirl the batter and cream cheese mixture by using a toothpick and then bake for 10 to 12 minutes until muffins have turned firm.

7. Serve and enjoy!

Nutrition: 261 Calories 23g Fats 7g Protein

Berries in Yogurt Cream

Preparation Time: 65 minutes

Cooking Time: 0 minutes

Servings: 2

Ingredients:

- 1-ounce blackberries
- 1-ounce raspberry
- 2 tbsp. erythritol sweetener
- 4 oz. yogurt
- 4 oz. whipping cream

Directions:

1. Take a medium bowl, place yogurt in it, and then whisk in cream.
2. Sprinkle sweetener over yogurt mixture, don't stir, cover the bowl with a lid, and then refrigerate for 1 hour.
3. When ready to serve, stir the yogurt mixture, divide it evenly between two bowls, top with berries, and then serve and enjoy!

Nutrition: 245 Calories 22g Fats 4g Protein

Pumpkin Pie Mug Cake

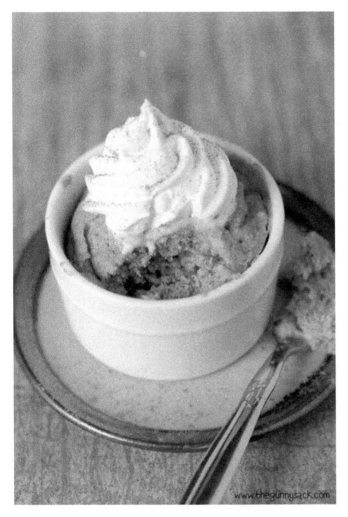

Preparation Time: 5 minutes

Cooking Time: 2 minutes

Servings: 2

Ingredients:

- 2 tbsp. coconut flour

- 1 tsp sour cream
- 2 tbsp. whipping cream
- 2 eggs
- ¼ cup pumpkin puree

Others:

- 2 tbsp. erythritol sweetener
- 1/3 tsp cinnamon
- ¼ tsp baking soda

Directions:

1. Take a small bowl, place cream in it, and then beat in sweetener until well combined.

2. Cover the bowl, let it chill in the refrigerator for 30 minutes, then beat in eggs and pumpkin puree and stir in remaining ingredients until incorporated and smooth.

3. Divide the batter between two coffee mugs greased with oil and then microwave for 2 minutes until thoroughly cooked.

4. Serve and enjoy!

Nutrition: 181 Calories 12g Fats 9g Protein

Chocolate and Strawberry Crepe

Preparation Time: 5 minutes

Cooking Time: 5 minutes

Servings: 2

Ingredients:

- 1 1/3 tbsp. coconut flour
- 1 tsp of cocoa powder
- ¼ tsp flaxseed
- 1 egg
- 2 ¾ tbsp. coconut milk, unsweetened
- 2 tsp avocado oil
- 1/8 tsp baking powder
- 2 oz. strawberry, sliced

Directions:

1. Take a medium bowl, place flour in it, and then stir in cocoa powder, baking powder, and flaxseed in it until mixed.
2. Add egg and milk and then whisk until smooth.
3. Take a medium skillet pan, place it over medium heat, add 1 tsp oil and when hot, pour in half of the batter, spread it evenly, and then cook for 1 minute per side until firm.

4. Transfer crepe to a plate, add remaining oil and cook another crepe by using the remaining batter.

5. When done, fill crepes with strawberries, fold them and then serve and enjoy!

Nutrition: 120 Calories 9g Fats 4g Protein

CONCLUSION

The world is constantly changing, and the possibilities to eat out may change from one day to another.

This book reveals the secret recipes of America's most famous meals, and you can now create these delicious dishes at home, yourself. With the recipes in this book, you will be able to make your favorite restaurant or fast-food meals at home, making the whole family happy, while you save a lot of money. This copycat recipe book is a great gift for any occasion, and it will be appreciated by anyone who is eager to learn about the secrets of cooking delicious restaurant meals in the comfort of their own home. From now on, you will be able to enjoy the taste of famous dishes from your favorite restaurants and fast-food chains at home.

Family meals have always been a big deal at our house. There's just nothing quite like getting your friends and loved ones together in the dining room to enjoy a tasty, piping hot home cooked meal. I get that some folks love eating out, but for me, you just can't beat a home cooked meal when it comes to cost, health, and really the whole experience! But just like anyone else, I have my favorite foods that I enjoy time to time from restaurants.

My experiencing trying to create "copycat" recipes from restaurants began years ago in earnest when I attempted to replicate the Big Mac sauce my kids loved so much. Turns out there was a little more to it than just opening a bottle of Thousand Islands dressings.

I had fun creating these recipes and, hopefully, you have been able to choose one to create; for me, all of them are tempting, so it's difficult to decide which one to make first. My strategy would be to pick one recipe for breakfast, one for lunch, one for a snack, and dinner every day. If you follow this recipe book and create the dishes described in it, your family will be amazed at your new cooking skills, and they will appreciate eating homemade food rather than always going to restaurants. I would like to thank you for investing your valuable time in reading my book; I am sure that it will be an easy-to-use and helpful tool in your kitchen.

You can entertain your friends and throw a house party with all the good meals from this book, but be careful because you might have them coming back often. My book of copycat recipes is not just for beginners, but also for experienced cooks who want to challenge themselves and have fun in the kitchen. I hope that you enjoy cooking these recipes, as well as eating them, and I wish you good appetite and a lot of fun!

If you have enjoyed this book, please leave me a review. For me, there is no greater reward than your satisfaction.

Leave me a comment if I miss any of your favorite restaurant's or brand's meals, so I can collect me

readers' favorites and create a Copycat Recipes part 2 for you soon.

CPSIA information can be obtained
at www.ICGtesting.com
Printed in the USA
BVHW052029120421
604748BV00001B/100